SURVIVING BREAST CANCER:

How To Deal With Breast Cancer

Dr. Bobby Franklin

DEDICATION

This book is dedicated to people battling cancer and to those who have died from this deadly illness. My thoughts are with their families and loved ones. Together we can win this battle against cancer.

TABLE OF CONTENT

INTRODUCTION

Breast cancers arise in the lining cells (epithelium) of the ducts (85%) or lobules (15%) in the glandular tissue of the breast. Initially, the cancerous increase is limited to the duct or lobule ("in situ") the place it generally causes no signs and symptoms and is minimally workable for spread (metastasis).

Over time, these cancers may additionally develop and invade the surrounding breast tissue (invasive breast cancer) and then spread to the nearby lymph nodes (regional metastasis) or different organs in the physique (distant metastasis). If a girl dies from breast cancer, it is because of large metastasis.

Breast cancer therapy can be exceedingly effective, especially when the sickness is recognized early. Treatment of breast cancer frequently consists of an aggregate of surgical removal, radiation remedy, and medication (hormonal therapy, chemotherapy, and/or focused biological therapy) to deal with microscopic cancer that has to unfold from the breast tumor via the blood. Such treatment can stop most cancers from booming and spreading, thereby saving lives.

Who Is At Risk?
Breast cancer is no longer a transmissible or infectious disease. Unlike some cancers that have infection-related causes, such as human papillomavirus (HPV) infection and cervical cancer, there are no recognized viral or bacterial infections linked to the development of breast cancer.

Approximately 1/2 of breast cancers increase in ladies who have no identifiable breast. Most cancers threaten components other than gender (female) and age (over 40 years). Certain factors make bigger the hazard of breast most cancers together with growing age, obesity, unsafe use of alcohol, family history of breast cancer, records of radiation exposure, reproductive history (such as the age that menstrual periods started and age at first pregnancy), tobacco use and postmenopausal hormone therapy.

Behavioral selections and related interventions that decrease the risk of breast most cancers include:

- Prolonged breastfeeding;
- Regular bodily activity;
- Weight control;
- Avoidance of hazardous use of alcohol;
- Avoidance of exposure to tobacco smoke;
- Avoidance of prolonged use of hormones; and
- Avoidance of excessive radiation exposure.

Unfortunately, even if all of the doubtlessly modifiable hazard factors ought to be controlled, this would solely limit the chance of growing breast cancer to at most 30%.

The female gender is the strongest breast cancer hazard factor. Approximately 0.5-1% of breast cancers take place in men. The remedy of breast cancers in men follows the identical principles of administration as for women.

Family records of breast cancer will increase the danger of breast cancer, but the majority of girls recognized with breast cancer do not now have a regarded household history of the disease. Lack of a recognized family history does no longer necessarily mean that a lady is at reduced risk.

Certain inherited "high penetrance" gene mutations greatly increase the breast most cancers risk, the most dominant being mutations in the genes BRCA1, BRCA2, and PALB-2. Women observed to have mutations in these primary genes should reflect on consideration of danger reduction strategies such as surgical elimination of both breasts. Consideration of such a distinctly invasive strategy solely worries a very confined wide variety of women, ought to be cautiously evaluated thinking about all preferences, and ought to no longer be rushed.

Scope Of The Problem.

In 2020, there will be 2.3 million ladies diagnosed with breast cancer and 685 zero deaths globally. As of 2020, there were 7.8 million ladies alive who have been diagnosed with breast cancer in the previous 5 years, making it the world's most accepted cancer. There are greater misplaced disability-adjusted existence years (DALYs) by females to breast cancers globally than any other type of cancer. Breast cancer takes place in each and every country of the world in girls at any age after puberty however with growing costs in later life.

Breast cancer mortality changed little from the Nineteen Thirties to the 1970s. Improvements in survival began in the Eighties in international locations with early detection programs blended with different modes of cure to eradicate invasive diseases.

Now let's comprehend the definition and full meaning of this deadly but curable disease.

CHAPTER 1

DEFINITION OF BREAST CANCER

Breast cancer is a sickness in which cells in the breast develop out of control. There are specific sorts of breast cancer.

Breast cancers happen when cells in your breast grow and divide in an uncontrolled way, creating a mass of tissue referred to as a tumor. Signs of breast cancer can consist of feeling a lump in your breast, experiencing a change in the dimension of your breast, and seeing changes to the pores and skin on your breasts. Mammograms can assist with early detection.

Breast most cancers can start in extraordinary components of the breast. A breast is made up of three important parts: lobules, ducts, and connective tissue. The lobules are the glands that produce milk. The ducts are tubes that carry milk to the nipple. The connective tissue (which consists of fibrous and fatty tissue) surrounds and holds the whole thing together. Most breast cancers begin in the ducts or lobules.

Breast cancer can spread to the backyard via blood vessels and lymph vessels. When breast cancer spreads to different components of the body, it is stated to have metastasized.

It's necessary to understand that most breast lumps are benign and no longer most cancers (malignant).

Non-cancer breast tumors are abnormal growths, however, they no longer unfold outdoors of the breast. They are now not life-threatening, but some kinds of benign breast lumps can expand a woman's risk of getting breast cancer. Any breast lump or trade wants to be checked by using a healthcare professional to locate out if it is benign or malignant (cancer) and if it might have an effect on your future most cancers risk.

Where Breast Cancers Start.

Breast cancers can start from different parts of the breast. The breast is an organ that sits on the pinnacle of the upper ribs and chest muscles. There is a left and right breast and each one has common glands, ducts, and fatty tissue. In women, the breast makes and delivers milk to feed newborns and infants. The amount of fatty tissue in the breast determines the size of each breast.

Breast cancers originate in your breast tissue. It occurs when breast cells mutate (change) and develop out of control, developing a mass of tissue (tumor). Like other cancers, breast cancer can invade and grow into the tissue surrounding your breast. It can additionally travel to other parts of your body and shape new tumors. When this happens, it's referred to as metastasis.

The Breast Has Distinct Parts:

Lobules are the glands that make breast milk. Cancers that start right here are referred to as lobular cancers.

Ducts are small canals that come out from the lobules and elevate the milk to the nipple. This is the most common location for breast cancer to start. Cancers that start right here are called ductal cancers.

The nipple is the opening in the skin of the breast where the ducts come collectively and turn into larger ducts so the milk can leave the breast. The nipple is surrounded with the aid of barely darker thicker pores and skin known as the areola. A much less frequent kind of breast cancer called Paget disorder of the breast can start in the nipple.

The fat and connective tissue (stroma) encompass the ducts and lobules and help keep them in place. A much less common kind of breast cancer called phyllodes tumor can begin in the stroma.

Blood vessels and lymph vessels are also located in every breast.

Angiosarcoma is a less frequent kind of breast cancer that can begin in the lining of these vessels. The lymph system is described below.

A small number of cancers begin in different tissues of the breast. These cancers are called sarcomas and lymphomas and are now not absolutely thought of as breast cancers.

How Breast Cancers Spread.
Breast cancers can unfold when the cancer cells get into the blood or lymph device and then are carried to other parts of the body.

The lymph (or lymphatic) system is a part of your body's immune system. It is a network of lymph nodes (small, bean-sized glands), ducts or vessels, and organs that work collectively to collect and carry clear lymph fluid through the body tissues to the blood. The clear lymph fluid inner the lymph vessels carry tissue by-products and waste material, as properly as immune system cells.

The lymph vessels carry lymph fluid away from the breast. In the case of breast cancer, most cancer cells can enter those lymph vessels and begin to grow in lymph nodes. Most of the lymph vessels of the breast drain into:

- Lymph nodes under the arm (axillary lymph nodes)
- Lymph nodes interior of the chest close to the breastbone (internal mammary lymph nodes)
- Lymph nodes around the collar bone (supraclavicular [above the collar bone] and infraclavicular [below the collar bone] lymph nodes)

If cancer cells have unfolded to your lymph nodes, there is a higher danger that the cells should have traveled through the lymph system and spread (metastasized) to other components of your body. Still, no longer all girls with most cancer cells in their lymph nodes boost metastases, and some girls with not most cancer cells in their lymph nodes might increase metastases later.

Who Is Mainly Affected By Breast Cancer?
Breast cancers are one of the most frequent cancers among women, 2nd solely to skin cancer. It's most likely to have an effect on ladies over the age of 50.

Though rare, guys can also have advanced breast cancer. Approximately 2,600 guys suffer male breast cancer each and every year in the United States, making up less than 1% of all cases.

Transgender women are more likely to advance breast cancers in contrast to cisgender men. Additionally, transgender men are much less likely to have advanced breast cancer in contrast to cisgender women.

What Age Does Breast Cancer Occur?

Breast cancers are most often identified in adults over the age of 50, however, it can take place at any age.

What Race Is Most Affected By Breast Cancer?

Overall, women who are non-Hispanic white have a barely higher hazard of developing breast cancer than females of any different race or ethnicity. Women who are non-Hispanic Black are nearly as likely as non-Hispanic white females to increase the disease. Statistically, ladies who are Asian, Hispanic, or Native American are the least probable to develop breast cancer.

How Frequent Is Breast Cancer?

In the United States, breast cancer is the second-leading motive of most cancer deaths in women, after lung cancer. It's additionally the main motive of most cancers demise among females a long time 35 to 54.

CHAPTER 2

TYPES OF BREAST CANCER

There are many exceptional sorts of breast cancers described via the place in the breast they commence to grow, how lots they have grown or spread, and sure features that influence how most cancers behave. The type of breast most cancers you've been diagnosed with will help you and your medical doctor decide on the nice treatment choices for you.

In this chapter, you will learn the one-of-a-kind types of breast cancer, the molecular subtypes of breast cancer, male breast cancer, and cancerous phyllodes tumors of the breast.

Invasive Breast Cancer.

When breast cancer is called invasive (or infiltrating), potentially it has to unfold into the surrounding breast tissue. The two most common kinds of invasive breast cancers are described by where in the breast they commence growing:

Invasive ductal carcinoma (IDC) is invasive breast cancer that starts in the milk ducts, the tubes that carry milk from the lobules to the nipple. It is the most common kind of breast cancer; about 80% of all breast cancers are invasive ductal carcinomas.

Invasive lobular carcinoma (ILC) is an invasive breast cancer that starts evolving in the lobules, the glands in the breast that produce milk. It is the 2nd most common type of breast cancer; about 10% of all invasive breast cancers are invasive lobular carcinomas.

Some types of invasive breast cancer have facets that affect how they boost and how they are treated:

Triple-negative breast cancer is an aggressive type of invasive breast cancer that checks poor for estrogen receptors and progesterone receptors and doesn't have more HER2 proteins. Triple terrible breast cancer now does not have any of the three receptors typically located on breast cancer cells (estrogen, progesterone, and HER2).

Around 15 percent of breast cancers are triple poor and chemotherapy is commonly recommended for these cancers. Targeted treatments and the function of immunotherapies are being actively studied in the treatment of triple-negative breast cancers. Immunotherapy medicines work by assisting the immune device to work harder and higher to fight cancer cells.

Inflammatory breast cancer is an uncommon and aggressive kind of invasive breast cancer that impacts the blood vessels in the skin and/or lymphatic vessels of the breast. This causes the breast to turn out to be pink and inflamed. About

1% of all breast cancers in the United States are inflammatory breast cancer.

Her2-Positive Breast Cancer.
HER2-positive breast cancer cells have lots of the protein known as human epidermal boom element receptor two on the surface of most cancer cells in contrast with ordinary cells. These excess HER2 receptors promote the boom of most cancer cells. HER2-positive breast cancer can also be either hormone receptor high-quality or negative. Around 20% of breast cancers are HER2-positive.

There are a variety of high-quality centered therapies to treat HER2-effective breast cancers. The targeted therapies are designed to target unique characteristics of the cancer cells such as the HER2 protein, stopping the cancer cells from dividing and growing. The drug trastuzumab is the most often used centered remedy for HER2-positive breast cancer. Most human beings with HER2-positive breast cancer will have focused remedies along with different treatments consisting of surgery, chemotherapy, and/or radiotherapy. They may additionally be encouraged hormone-blocking therapy if the cancer is additionally hormone receptor-positive.

Metastatic breast cancer, also called stage IV breast cancer, is invasive breast cancer that has spread (metastasized) to components of the body away from the breast, such as the bones, liver, lungs, or brain. Breast cancer can come lower back in any other phase of the body months or years after the original treatment (called a metastatic recurrence), but some human beings are in the beginning identified with metastatic sickness (called de novo metastatic breast cancer).

Recurrent breast cancer is invasive breast cancer that has come again months or years after treatment. Breast cancers can recur in the same breast (local recurrence), close to lymph nodes in the armpit or collarbone (regional recurrence), or in every other section of the body, (metastatic or far-off recurrence).

Male breast cancer is rare, but it does happen. Fewer than 1% of all breast cancers are diagnosed in men. Most male breast cancers are invasive ductal carcinomas.

Paget disorder of the breast is a rare form of breast cancer where most cancer cells acquire in or around the nipple.

There are also five important molecular subtypes of invasive breast cancer primarily based on the genes in the cancer tumor. The molecular subtype of breast cancers can affect how most cancers are treated.

Non-invasive Breast Cancer.
When breast cancer is known as non-invasive (or in situ) it's ability no longer unfolds beyond the breast tissue the place it started. Non-invasive breast cancers are additionally referred to as precancers. There are two foremost sorts of non-invasive breast cancer:

Ductal carcinoma in situ (DCIS), is non-invasive breast cancer that has not unfolded outdoors in the milk ducts the place they started. DCIS isn't existence-threatening, but is viewed as a precursor to invasive breast cancer and increases the risk of developing invasive breast cancers later in life. About 16% of all breast cancer diagnoses are DCIS.

Lobular carcinoma in situ (LCIS), is non-invasive breast cancer that has not spread outside the lobules where it started. Despite its name, LCIS is a benign breast circumstance and is now not a true breast cancer.

Cancerous Phyllodes Tumors Of The Breast.
Phyllodes tumors of the breast are rare and make up fewer than 1% of all breast tumors. Most phyllodes tumors are benign (not cancerous), but about 25% are cancerous. Phyllodes tumors tend to grow quickly, however, they hardly ever spread backyard the breast. Phyllodes tumors develop in the breast's connective tissue or stroma (the tissue that holds the whole thing

collectively inside the breast) i.e. outdoor the ducts and lobules of the breast.

Other Rare Breast Cancers.
There are additionally different types of very rare breast cancers such as metaplastic, medullary, and mucinous breast cancer.

Locally Superior Breast Cancer.
Locally superior breast cancer is an invasive breast cancers that are 5cm or larger or have spread beyond the breast to other nearby areas such as the skin, chest wall, or muscle and may have massive local lymph node involvement.

CHAPTER 3

CAUSES OF BREAST CANCER

Breast cancers originate in breast tissue. It's brought about with the aid of changes, or mutations, in breast cell phone DNA. These mutations reason cells to develop abnormally and divide more quickly than healthy cells do. The extraordinary cells accumulate, forming a malignant breast mass, also regarded as a lump.

Your immune gadget may additionally be able to effectively combat some abnormal cells. but the ones that continue to grow might also spread, or metastasize, in the course of the breast to the lymph nodes or different parts of the body.

When breast cancer spreads, the malignant tumors it motives in other places are nevertheless referred to as breast cancer. What precisely triggers DNA modifications in breast cells isn't clear. Two humans can have equal or similar hazard factors, however solely one may improve breast cancer.

Breast cancers are the most common kind of cancer among females. It is caused with the aid of the unusual division of cells and subsequent formation of a mass of tissue known as a tumor. Understanding the causes of breast cancer enables you to become aware of doable risk factors, which can lead to early detection and treatment.

Gender And Age.
Aging girls are extra in all likelihood than guys to increase breast cancer. The danger of developing breast cancer will increase with age. The condition is most common in ladies over age 50 who have been via menopause. About 8 out of 10 cases of breast cancer appear in women over 50.

Genetics.

It is estimated that 5 to 10 percent of breast cancers are linked to inherited gene mutations.

Breast most cancers gene 1 (BRCA1) and breast cancer gene 2 (BRCA2) are the most frequent breast most cancers genes. They are tumor suppressor genes that commonly have the job of controlling cell phone boom and cellphone death. Changes to their shape may motivate most cancer tumors to grow. Doctors may additionally endorse that sufferers with a familial record of breast cancer undergo blood assessments to perceive feasible BRCA mutations.

The PTEN gene helps manage phone increase and death. Damage to this gene creates a greater danger for each cancerous and noncancerous breast tumor. The TP53 gene tells cells to make a protein referred to as p53, which helps end the increase of ordinary cells. Changes in TP53 cause an extended threat of breast cancer, leukemia, Genius tumors, and childhood sarcomas. Less than 1 percent of all breast cancer is thought to be related to this gene.

History Of Breast Conditions.

Previous breast conditions, especially lobular carcinoma in situ (LCIS) or odd breast hyperplasia, might also be one of the motives for breast cancer. Also, a female whose breasts have vast areas of dense tissue on mammograms is a multiplied threat for breast cancer.

Patients who have had cancer in one breast are at an elevated risk to increase most cancers in the other breast. If you have a close family who has had breast cancer or ovarian cancer, you may also have a greater risk of developing breast cancer.

However, because breast cancer is the most common cancer in women, it can appear in greater than one family member by chance. Most instances of breast cancer do not run in families, however, genes acknowledged as BRCA1 and BRCA2 can make your hazard of developing each breast and ovarian cancer bigger. These genes can be surpassed by a guardian of their child.

The genes TP53 and CHEK2, are also related to an elevated hazard of breast cancer.

Speak to a GP if breast or ovarian cancer runs in your household and you are involved you may additionally get it too. They may also refer you for an NHS genetic test, which will inform you if you have inherited one of the cancer-risk genes.

Previous Breast Cancers Or Lump.
If you have before had breast cancers or early non-invasive cancers mobile phone modifications in breast ducts, you have a higher risk of growing it again, both in your different breast or in the same breast. A benign breast lump does not now imply you have breast cancer, however sure types of breast lumps may also slightly enlarge your threat of creating cancer.

Some benign changes in your breast tissue, such as cells growing abnormally in ducts (atypical ductal hyperplasia), or peculiar cells internal to your breast lobes (lobular carcinoma in situ), can make getting breast cancer more likely.

Dense Breast Tissue.
Your breasts are made up of thousands of tiny glands (lobules) that produce milk. This glandular tissue incorporates greater attention to breast cells than different breast tissue, making it denser.

Women with dense breast tissue can also have a greater hazard of growing breast cancer as there are extra cells that can turn out to be cancerous. Dense breast tissue can additionally make a breast scan (mammogram) difficult to read, as any lumps or areas of unusual tissue are tougher to see.

Younger girls tend to have dense breasts. As you get older, the quantity of glandular tissue in your breasts decreases and is replaced by using fat, so your breasts turn out to be much less dense.

Exposure To Estrogen.
The lady hormone estrogen can every so often stimulate breast cancer cells and motivate them to grow.

The ovaries, the place your eggs are stored, start to produce estrogen when you start puberty, to regulate your periods. Your chance of growing breast cancers may additionally rise slightly with the quantity of estrogen your body is uncovered to.

For example, if you started out having durations at a younger age and experienced menopause later than average, you will have been uncovered to estrogen over a longer period.

Identically, no longer having teens or having youngsters later in life may barely extend your threat of developing breast cancers because your publicity to estrogen is not interrupted by way of pregnancy.

Hormone Substitute Remedy (Hrt).
Hormone substitute therapy (HRT) is associated with an elevated danger of creating breast cancer.

All kinds of HRT can enlarge the hazard of breast cancer, without vaginal estrogen. There is no accelerated risk of breast cancer if you take HRT for much less than 1 year.

But if you take HRT for longer than 1 year, you have a higher chance of breast cancer than ladies who by no means use HRT. The elevated risk of breast cancer falls after you quit taking HRT, however, some accelerated chance stays for more than 10 years compared to women who have in no way used HRT.

Contraceptive Pill.
Research shows that females who take the contraceptive pill have a barely increased chance

of growing breast cancer. However, the risk starts to minimize as soon as you quit taking the pill, and your threat of breast cancer is back to normal every day 10 years after stopping.

Radiation Exposure.
Radiation treatments to the chest throughout youth or young adulthood can be one of the motives for breast cancer.

Certain clinical approaches that use radiation, such as X-rays and CT scans, may barely increase your risk of growing breast cancer.

If you had radiotherapy to your chest area for Hodgkin lymphoma you need to have already obtained a letter from the Department of Health and Social Care inviting you for a session with a specialist to talk about the multiplied danger of creating breast cancer.

See your GP if you have not been contacted or if you have not attended a consultation. You're commonly entitled to have your breast checked with an MRI scan. If you currently want radiotherapy for Hodgkin lymphoma, your specialist discusses the risk of breast cancer earlier than your therapy begins.

Obesity.
Being obese will increase the chance of breast cancer.
Giving delivery to a first child at an older age. Women who have their first infant after age 30 can also have a multiplied threat of breast cancer. If you have skilled menopause and are obese or obese, you may additionally be extra at threat of creating breast cancer.

This is thought to be linked to the amount of estrogen in your body, as being obese or chubby after menopause causes extra estrogen to be produced.

Beginning Menstruation At A Younger Age.
Beginning menstruation earlier than age 12 increases the danger of breast cancer.

Beginning Menopause At An Older Age.
Beginning menopause after age 55 increases the risk of breast cancer.

Pregnancy. Women who have by no means been pregnant are at an increased danger of creating breast cancer.

Post-menopausal hormone therapy. Estrogen and progesterone medicines taken to treat the symptoms of menopause may additionally expand the chance of breast cancer. Fortunately, the chance decreases when these medicinal drugs are discontinued.

Alcohol Use.
Drinking alcohol excessively will increase the danger of breast cancer. People who drink even small quantities of alcohol on a normal foundation have a larger threat of getting breast cancer than humans who do not now drink alcohol at all. The greater alcohol you drink, the more your hazard of getting breast cancer increases.

Diethylstilbestrol (DES) Exposure. Women who take this medicine while pregnant to lower the chance of miscarriage are at greater risk. Women whose moms took DES all through pregnancy can also have a greater risk.

Newly recognized breast cancer patients, especially those who have identified hazard factors, need to be tested for HER2 breast cancer. Identifying HER2 breast cancer early may also extend the chances of therapy success.

CHAPTER 4

RISK FACTORS OF BREAST CANCER

Studies have proven that your risk for breast cancer is due to an aggregate of factors. The foremost factors that affect your danger include being a lady and getting older. Most breast cancers are discovered in females who are 50 years old or older.

Some girls will get breast cancer even besides any different chance elements that they are aware of. Having a danger issue does not mean you will get the disease, and no longer all threat elements have an identical effect. Most ladies have some chance factors, however, most ladies do not get breast cancer. If you have breast cancer danger factors, discuss with your physician about approaches you can lower your chance and about screening for breast cancer.

Risk Factors You Cannot Change.

Getting older. The risk of breast cancer will increase with age. Most breast cancers are recognized after age 50.

Race And Ethnicity.

Breast cancer is the most frequent cancer prognosis in women, other than skin cancer, regardless of race. White women are greater in all likelihood to increase breast cancer than Black women, but among women youthful than 45, the disease is more frequent in Black women than in White women. Black females are also more probable to die from the disease. Reasons for survival differences might also encompass differences in biology, other fitness conditions, and socioeconomic factors affecting access to, and use of, medical care.

Women of Ashkenazi or Eastern European Jewish heritage additionally have an improved hazard of breast cancers due to the fact they can also be greater, probably to have inherited a BRCA1 gene mutation. Breast cancers are least generally recognized in Hispanic, Asian/Pacific Islander, and American Indian/Alaska Native women. Both Black ladies and Hispanic ladies are extra probable to be identified with larger tumors and later-stage cancer than White women. However, Hispanic ladies commonly have better survival fees than White women. Breast cancer diagnoses have been increasing in 2nd generation Asian/Pacific Islander and Hispanic girls for uncertain reasons. However, the amplification is possibly related to adjustments in the food plan and way of life associated with dwelling in the United States.

Genetic Mutations.

Women who have inherited adjustments (mutations) to positive genes, such as BRCA1 and BRCA2, are at higher risk of breast and ovarian cancer.

There are quite a few inherited genetic mutations linked with a multiplied chance of breast cancer, as properly as other kinds of cancer. BRCA1 or BRCA2 are the most commonly recognized genes linked to breast cancer. Mutations in these genes are linked to an improved chance of breast and ovarian cancers, as well as different sorts of cancer. Male breast cancer, as well as the danger of prostate cancer and other cancers, is additionally elevated if there is a mutation in 1 of these genes.

Other gene mutations or hereditary conditions can enlarge a person's threat of breast cancer. They are much less common than BRCA1 or BRCA2, and they do not extend the chance of breast cancer as much. Some of these genes and syndromes are:

- Lynch syndrome, linked with the MLH1, MSH2, MSH6, and PMS2 genes
- Cowden syndrome (CS), linked with the PTEN gene

- Li-Fraumeni syndrome (LFS), linked with the TP53 gene
- Peutz-Jeghers syndrome (PJS), linked with the STK11 gene
- Ataxia telangiectasia (A-T), linked with the ATM gene
- Hereditary diffuse gastric cancer, linked with the CDH1 gene
- PALB2 gene
- CHEK2 gene

There are additionally different genes that can also cause an extended risk of breast cancer. More research is needed to recognize how they expand a person's risk. For example, an individual can inherit a gene mutation but now not increase breast cancer. Research is additionally ongoing to find other genes that may also affect breast cancer risk.

Genetic checking through blood exams is reachable to take a look at for acknowledged mutations in BRCA1 and BRCA2 genes and different genes linked with hereditary syndromes. Ask your physician if genetic checking out is encouraged for you. Your doctor might also suggest a check called a "panel test." A panel takes a look at appearances of mutations in countless distinctive genes at identical times. There are specific panel tests your physician can recommend. However, these tests are no longer recommended for everyone, and it is endorsed that people acquire terrific genetic counseling earlier than the present process checking out to make sure they have the right to take a look at performance, and so they understand the results of the tests.

There are also tests that a character can request immediately from a trying-out business enterprise that does not require a doctor's order. These are usually completed with the aid of using a package despatched thru the mail. If you choose to have one of these exams performed, you need to discuss it with your health practitioner first, as some assessments only test a restricted quantity of genes. This skill might also supply incomplete information, and you may also need a specific check performed to take a look at all the genes that may additionally be essential for you primarily based on your family history. In addition, you may additionally need to repeat checking out to affirm that the effects are correct.

If a person learns they have a genetic mutation, there may additionally be steps they can take to lower their danger of breast and ovarian cancers (see "Prevention," below). They may also need an extraordinary breast cancer screening schedule than the well-known population, such as having distinctive sorts of checks or beginning screening at a younger age. In addition, they may additionally want specific sorts of screening exams for other cancers, such as having a colonoscopy at a youthful age to observe colorectal cancer.

Reproductive History.
Starting menstrual periods before age 12 and beginning menopause after age fifty-five expose

females to hormones longer, raising their hazard of getting breast cancer.

This is due to the fact the breast cells have been uncovered to estrogen and progesterone for a longer time. Estrogen and progesterone are hormones that manipulate the development of secondary sex characteristics, such as breast development, and pregnancy. The production of estrogen and progesterone decreases with age, with a steep minimization around menopause. Longer publicity of these hormones will increase breast cancer risk.

Having Dense Breasts.
Dense breasts have extra connective tissue than fatty tissue, which can every so often make it hard to see tumors on a mammogram. Women with dense breasts are more likely to get breast cancer.

Dense breast tissue may also make it more difficult to notice a tumor on fashionable imaging tests, such as mammography. Having dense breast tissue usually means you have greater milk glands, milk ducts, and supportive tissue in the breast than fatty tissue. On a mammogram, it can be more difficult to distinguish a tumor from ordinary history tissue when the tissue is dense.

Dense breast tissue is a measure used to describe mammogram pix as adverse to how the breast feels. Breast density generally decreases with age. Some states require that mammogram outcomes include facts about breast density if the outcomes exhibit that an individual has dense breast tissue. However, at this time, there are no specific screening suggestions for humans with dense breasts.

Personal history of breast cancer or positive non-cancerous breast diseases. Women who have had breast most cancers are extra probably to get breast most cancers a 2nd time. Some non-cancerous breast illnesses such as atypical hyperplasia or lobular carcinoma in situ are associated with a higher danger of getting breast cancer.

Family History Of Breast Or Ovarian Cancer.
A woman's hazard for breast cancer is greater if she has a mother, sister, or daughter (first-degree relative) or a couple of family contributors on both her mother's or father's facet of the family who has had breast or ovarian cancer. Having a first-degree male relative with breast cancer also raises a woman's risk.

BRCA1 and BRCA2 gene mutations substantially increase the risk of ovarian cancer and breast cancer. Therefore, a character diagnosed with hereditary ovarian cancers prompted through a BRCA gene mutation has an increased risk of breast cancer as well. Women with breast cancers who did not inherit a BRCA1 or BRCA2 mutation commonly do now not have a higher chance of ovarian cancer.

Breast cancer may additionally run in the family in any of these situations:

- 1 or greater women are recognized with breast cancer at age forty-five or younger
- 1 or greater ladies are diagnosed with breast cancer before age 50 with an extra family history of cancer, such as ovarian cancer, metastatic prostate cancer, and pancreatic cancer
- There are breast and/or ovarian cancers in a couple of generations on 1 facet of the family, such as having a grandmother and an aunt on the father's side of the family who were both recognized with 1 of these cancers
- A woman in the family is identified with a second breast cancer in the equal or the different breast or has both breast and ovarian cancer
- A male relative is diagnosed with breast cancer

Having Ashkenazi Jewish Ancestry.

It is vital to talk with your doctor if your household has experienced any of the above situations. It could be a signal that your household includes an inherited breast cancer genetic mutation, such as BRCA1 or BRCA2.

When looking at family history, it's additionally important to consider your father's facet of the family. Your father's aspect is equally important as your mother's side in finding out your threat for creating breast cancer.

Previous Treatment In The Use Of Radiation Therapy.
Women who had radiation therapy to the chest or breasts (for instance, cure of Hodgkin's lymphoma) before age 30 have a higher danger of getting breast cancer later in life.

Exposure to the drug diethylstilbestrol (DES).
DES was once given to some pregnant girls in the United States between 1940 and 1971 to stop miscarriage. Women who took DES, or whose mothers took DES whilst pregnant with them, have a greater hazard of getting breast cancer.

Risk Factors You Can Change.

Not Being Bodily Active.
Women who are no longer physically energetic have a higher risk of getting breast cancer.
Being overweight or having obesity after menopause. Older ladies who are obese or have obesity have a higher chance of getting breast cancer than those at a healthy weight.

Taking Hormones.
Some types of hormone replacement therapy (those that encompass estrogen and progesterone) taken in the course of menopause can raise the chance of breast cancer when taken for an extra five years.

Using hormone therapy with both estrogen and progestin after menopause, regularly referred to as postmenopausal hormone therapy or hormone alternative therapy, within the previous 5 years or for several years will increase the threat of breast cancer. The quantity of new breast cancers recognized has dropped extensively as there is now much less use of postmenopausal hormone therapy. However, women who have taken only estrogen, except those formerly receiving progestin, for up to 5 years (because they had their uterus eliminated for different reasons) appear to have a slight decrease chance of breast cancer.

Oral Contraceptives Or Delivery Manipulate Pills.

Some research suggests that oral contraceptives to stop being pregnant slightly enlarge the danger of breast cancer, whilst others have shown no hyperlink between the use of oral contraceptives and the improvement of breast cancer. Research on this subject matter is ongoing.

Reproductive History.

Having the first pregnancy after age 30 or if you've in no way had a full-term pregnancy brings a higher threat of breast cancer. Pregnancy may additionally help protect against breast cancer because it pushes breast cells into their ultimate phase of maturation. Breastfeeding, and having a full-term pregnancy can limit breast cancer risk.

Atypical Hyperplasia Of The Breast.
This prognosis will increase the danger of creating breast cancer in the future. It is characterized by abnormal, however no longer cancerous, cells determined in a biopsy of the breast.

Lobular Carcinoma In Situ (LCIS). LCIS refers to peculiar cells discovered in the lobules or glands of the breast. It is no longer considered cancer. However, LCIS in 1 breast will increase the danger of creating invasive breast cancers in both breasts in the future. If LCIS is observed at some stage in a biopsy, it might also be eliminated to check for other changes. Talk with your medical doctor about the best way to screen and deal with this condition.

Radiation Exposure At A Young Age.
Exposure to ionizing radiation at a younger age

may additionally amplify a woman's danger of breast cancer. For example, therapeutic radiation to the chest for Hodgkin lymphoma can also extend breast cancer hazard in each breast.

The very small quantity of radiation a character receives at some stage in a mammogram has now not been linked to an increased threat of breast cancer.

Drinking Alcohol.
Studies show that a woman's threat of breast cancer will increase with the more alcohol she drinks.

Studies suggest that having greater than 1 to 2 servings of alcohol, consisting of beer, wine, and spirits, per day raises the threat of breast cancer. It is recommended to limit your alcohol consumption to 3 to four servings per week.

Food.
There is no reliable research that confirms that ingesting or keeping off specific foods increases

the danger of developing breast cancer or having cancer come again after treatment. However, ingesting more fruits and greens and less animal fat is linked with many health benefits, together with a slight reduction in the risk of breast cancer.

Research suggests that other elements such as smoking, being uncovered to chemicals that can cause cancer, and modifications in other hormones due to night shift working additionally may additionally amplify breast cancer risk. For humans with a private record of breast most cancers or a sturdy family history of breast cancer, other methods of identifying their chance of breast most cancers may additionally work better. People with a sturdy family record of breast cancer risk ought to consider talking to a genetic counselor.

It is vital to speak with your doctor about how to estimate your non-public hazard of breast cancer and to talk about risk-reducing or prevention options.

CHAPTER 5

SYMPTOMS OF BREAST CANCER

Early Symptoms Of Breast Cancer.
Early on, a person may additionally be aware of a change in their breast when they operate a monthly breast exam or when minor unusual pain doesn't appear to go away.

Many types of breast cancer exist and have special symptoms. Signs differ widely, and some humans do not have early signs at all. You may observe adjustments in your breasts whilst doing day-to-day activities such as taking a shower. The ACS recommends if you have an average threat of breast cancer start regular screening mammograms between a long time of 45–54 (but you can start as early as 40).

Here are some common early symptoms of breast cancer. Trust your gut, and in no way hesitate to speak to a healthcare provider.

A New Breast Lump.
A lump in the breast, on occasion as little as a pea, is the most frequent early signal of breast cancer.

Most breast lumps are not cancerous. Lumps that aren't most cancers are referred to as benign lumps.

Most benign breast lumps are:

- Areas of normal lumpiness that are more apparent just before a period
- Cysts – sacs of fluid in the breast tissue, which are pretty common
- Fibroadenoma – a collection of fibrous glandular tissue (these are common in younger women, for example under 30)

That said, again most breast lumps are not cancer. If you discover one:

- You may also have a non-cancerous breast cyst—a lump filled with fluid—or a fibrocystic condition
- Cancerous lumps are extra in all likely to be painless and with irregular edges
- Cancerous lumps can on occasion be "soft, round, tender, or even painful"
- A lump in the armpit can additionally be a signal of concern.

A Lump Or Swelling In Your Armpit.
You can't generally feel the lymph glands in your body. But they often grow to be swollen when you have contamination or cold, along with the lymph nodes in the armpit.

A less frequent motive of swollen lymph glands or lump in the armpit is breast cancer that has spread to this area.

Change In Size, Shape, Or Feel Of Your Breast.

Most cancers might motivate your breast to appear higher or have a one-of-a-kind structure than usual, it may experience different.

Many wholesome females find that their breasts feel lumpy and gentle simply earlier than their period.

It can assist to be breast aware. This means getting to understand the size, form, and feel of your breasts.

Some modifications in the breast are natural and can appear due to the fact of weight changes, aging, around your period, menopause, or during pregnancy. Hormonal medicines like start management drugs or menopausal hormone therapy can make breasts denser.

Sometimes, if you have breast cancer, you might also notice other changes before you can experience a lump. Forms of breast cancer, such as aggressive inflammatory breast cancer, may come beside any lumps. Early breast look modifications that should signal breast most cancers include:

- Swelling of all or phases of the breast
- Dimpling (the skin looking like an orange peel)—typically a symptom of inflammatory breast cancer
- Skin changes such as dryness, thickness, or flaking
- An indentation that doesn't go away when you take off your bra
- Sudden modifications in color
- Other changes in shape and measurement unexplained by using herbal or medication-related causes

Skin Changes.

Skin changes encompass puckering, dimpling, a rash, or redness of the pores and skin of the breast. Some people have a rash or redness of the nipple and the surrounding skin.

The pores and skin might look like orange peel or the texture would possibly sense differently. This can be prompted by different breast conditions. But get your doctor to take a look at something that is now not regular for you.

Nipple Changes.
The nipple or nipple area can additionally be affected. Nipple adjustments that might also be a breast most cancers symptom include:

- Inverted nipple, or nipple that turns inward: This can be a herbal change, though.
- Skin modifications in the nipple area: Changes include redness, dryness, crusting, or flaking.
- Discharge that isn't always breast milk, such as blood: This can additionally be induced using delivery control pills, medications, and infections
- Pain

Fluid Leaking From Your Nipple

Fluid leaking from a nipple in a female who is not pregnant or breastfeeding can be a sign of cancer. But other medical prerequisites can additionally purpose this.

Breast Thickening or Pain

Your breast may feel thicker, or you may additionally experience pain in phase or all of it. Both signs are often signs and symptoms of a much less serious condition—birth management drugs can also make breasts denser, and fibrosis (a common situation that causes lumps in the breast) can cause pain, mainly around a person's period.5 But talk to a healthcare provider to rule out cancer.

Other early signs of breast cancer to look for include:

- Changes in the structure of the nipple
- Breast pain that doesn't go away after your subsequent period
- A new lump that doesn't go away after your subsequent period

- Nipple discharge from one breast that's clear, red, brown, or yellow
- Unexplained redness, swelling, skin irritation, itchiness, or rash on the breast
- Swelling or a lump around the collarbone or below the arm
- A lump that's hard with irregular edges is extra, probably to be cancerous.

Later Signs And Symptoms Of Breast Cancer
Later signs and symptoms of breast most cancers include:

- Retraction, or inward turning of the nipple
- Enlargement of one breast
- Dimpling of the breast surface
- an existing lump that receives a bigger
- An "orange peel" texture to the skin
- Poor appetite
- Unintentional weight loss
- Enlarged lymph nodes in the armpit
- Visible veins on the breast

Having one or greater of these symptoms doesn't necessarily mean you have breast cancer. Nipple discharge, for example, can also be induced with the aid of an infection. See a doctor for a complete comparison if you experience any of these symptoms and symptoms.

Experiencing any of these modifications can be scary, but it is vital to have in mind that most don't seem to be due to breast cancer. And if you get a diagnosis, recognize there are many remedy preferences already available, with extra in the works. Just make certain to see a healthcare company ASAP—early analysis and treatment are vital for a better outcome.

CHAPTER 6

PREVENTION OF BREAST CANCER

These easy steps can assist lower the hazard of breast cancer. Not every one applies to every woman, however, as a whole, they can have a massive impact.

1. Keep Weight in Check

It's handy to pass due to the fact it gets said so often, however retaining a healthy weight is important for everyone. Being overweight can increase the threat of many unique cancers, including breast cancer, especially after menopause.

2. Be Physically Active

Exercise is as shut to a silver bullet for proper fitness as there is. Women who exercise for at least 30 minutes a day have a decreased danger of breast cancer. Regular exercise is additionally one of the excellent methods to help preserve weight in check.

I recommend:

- Getting a weekly total of one hundred fifty to 300 minutes of rather excessive activity (exercise that you can do while holding a conversation), or 75 to one hundred fifty minutes of lively activity, or a combination of the two
- Strength coaching and stretching to improve balance and flexibility about twice a week
- Limiting sedentary activities, such as observing TV

3. Eat Your Fruits & Vegetables – and Limit Alcohol (Zero is Best)

A healthful eating regimen can assist decrease the danger of breast cancer. Try to consume a whole lot of culmination and greens and restrict alcohol. Even low tiers of ingesting can increase the risk of breast cancer. And with different dangers of alcohol, now no longer consuming is the general quality desired for your fitness.

I endorse a plant-primarily based eating regimen wealthy in complete grains, greens, culmination, and beans. Incorporate brightly colored or strongly flavored veggies and culmination into your food regimen. Limit purple and processed meats, sugary liquids and sodas, and processed meals excessive in fats and starch.

4. Don't Smoke

On pinnacle of its many different fitness dangers, smoking causes at least 15 one-of-a-kind cancers – along with breast cancers. If you smoke, attempt to stop as quickly as possible. It's nearly by no means too past due to get advantages. You can do it. And getting assistance can double your possibility of quitting for good

5. Limit Or Avoid Alcohol

Any quantity of alcohol will increase your threat of breast cancer. Research suggests that more alcohol intake is connected to better breast cancer risk. Avoiding alcohol is ideal, however, in case you do pick out to devour it, restrict yourself to no extra than 3 to 5 servings in keeping with the week.

6. Breastfeed, If Possible

Breastfeeding for a complete 12 months or extra (mixed for all children) lowers the danger of breast cancer. It additionally has amazing fitness advantages for the child. For breastfeeding records or support, touch your pediatrician, health facility, or nearby fitness department.

7. Manage Stress

Although there may be no demonstrated hyperlink between pressure and extended breast most cancers chance, lowering pressure ranges possibly advantages ordinary fitness. Helpful practices consist of:

8. Deep Respiration And Meditation

- A regular workout that consists of stretching
- Taking breaks from information reviews and social media
- Seeking assistance from a psychologist, social employee, or expert counselor in case you face ongoing excessive degrees of strain.

9. Avoid Birth Control Pills, Particularly After Age 35 or If You Smoke

Birth manipulation tablets have both dangers and advantages. The more youthful a girl is, the decrease the dangers are. While ladies are taking delivery-managed tablets, they have a barely expanded danger of breast cancer. This danger is going away quickly, though, after preventing the pill.

The hazard of stroke and coronary heart assault is likewise extended at the same time as at the pill – in particular if a lady smokes. But long-time period use also can have critical advantages, like reducing the hazard of ovarian, colon, and uterine cancers. Birth management tablets additionally save you from undesirable pregnancy, so there's additionally plenty in their favor. If you're very involved in breast cancer, keeping off the beginning and manipulating tablets is one choice to decrease the threat.

10. Avoid Hormone Therapy for Menopause

Hormone remedies in menopause shouldn't be taken a long time to save you from persistent illnesses. Studies display its blended results on fitness, elevating the threat of a few sicknesses and reducing the threat of others. Whether estrogen is taken through itself or it's blended with progestin, hormones grow the danger of breast cancers. If girls do take hormone remedies throughout menopause, it has to be for the shortest time possible. The fine individual to speak to approximately the dangers and blessings of hormone remedies for menopause is your health practitioner.

11. Tamoxifen And Raloxifene For Women At High Risk

Although now no longer usually thought of as a "wholesome behavior," taking the medicine tamoxifen and raloxifene can significantly decrease the chance of breast cancers in girls at excessive danger of the disease. Approved via means of the FDA for breast cancer prevention, those effective tablets could have side effects, so they aren't proper for everyone. If you watched you're at the excessive chance, to speak to your physician to peer if those pills can be proper for you.

12. Find Out Your Family History

Women with a robust circle of relatives with records of most cancers can take unique steps to defend themselves. That's why it's key for ladies to realize their circle of relatives' records. You're in more danger when you have a mom or sister who had breast or ovarian cancers. This danger is even better in case your relative becomes recognized at an early age. Having more than one own circle of relatives members (inclusive of males) who had breast, ovarian, or prostate cancers additionally increases your chance. A physician or genetic counselor can assist explain your circle of relatives' records of the disease.

13. Don't Forget Mammograms

Breast cancer screening with mammography saves lives. It doesn't assist save you against most cancers, however, it could assist discover most cancers early while it's extra treatable.

Most ladies have to get one every year mammograms beginning at age 40.

Women at better risk for breast cancer might also additionally want to begin getting screened in advance. It's a quality to speak to a physician via way of means of age 30 approximately your chance and whether or not you'd benefit from in advance screening.

Because ordinary breast self-tests haven't been established to be beneficial, they aren't endorsed for screening. Still, understanding your breasts is key. Tell your physician properly in case you note any adjustments in how your breasts appear or feel.

For Sufferers At Excessive Hazard For Breast Cancers

If you face an expanded danger of breast cancer, you could take a few extra steps to lessen your chance. Consider the following:

Enhanced Screening

Breast cancer screening can not save breast cancers from growing, however, it may assist in coming across it in advance, while it is less difficult to deal with. Ask your gynecologist or number one care physician approximately a tailor-made screening program. This may also encompass extra or unique styles of imaging tests.

Tamoxifen

Tamoxifen, an anti-estrogen medication, has been used for many years to deal with breast cancer. A big look known as the Breast Cancer Prevention Trial observed that during wholesome girls without breast cancers, 5 years of tamoxifen use decreased the chance of growing it by about 50%.

To determine whether or not taking tamoxifen is proper for you, communicate with your medical doctor.

Prophylactic (Preventive) Mastectomy
Some sufferers with an excessive hazard of growing breast most cancers can also additionally select to have one or each breast surgically removed. These encompass sufferers who've:

- Mutations of the BRCA1 or BRCA2 genes
- A record of breast most cancers
- Several near-loved ones laid low with breast cancers
- A biopsy displaying lobular carcinoma in situ (a situation that could precede the improvement of invasive most cancers)

Even a notably professional doctor can not cast off all breast tissue from the chest, however, so a small percentage of sufferers who've preventive mastectomies nonetheless come to be growing breast cancers. The choice to have this surgical procedure takes an extremely good deal of meaning. Patients who do not forget this preventive approach must communicate with numerous docs beforehand, and weigh the scientific and emotional outcomes of the surgical operation in opposition to the advantages.

Some sufferers will also be applicants for prophylactic oophorectomy, or elimination of the ovaries, to lessen the breast most cancers threat.

CHAPTER 7

DIAGNOSIS

Doctors use many tests to find, or diagnose, breast cancer. They may additionally do checks to study if most cancers have spread to a part of the physique other than the breast and the lymph nodes underneath the arm. If cancer has spread, it is called metastasis. Doctors may additionally also do exams to study which redress ought to work best.

For most kinds of cancer, a biopsy is the sole sure way for the physician to comprehend if a region of the physique has cancer. In a biopsy, the health practitioner takes a small pattern of tissue for testing in a laboratory. If a biopsy is no longer possible, the physician may propose other exams that will help make a diagnosis.

How Breast Cancer Is Diagnosed

There are many checks used for diagnosing breast cancer. Not all tests described right here will be used for each person. Your doctor can also consider these elements when selecting a diagnostic test:

- The kind of cancer suspected
- Your symptoms and symptoms
- Your age and frequent health
- The consequences of the past medical tests

The collection of checks wished to evaluate a possible breast cancer commonly starts when a person or their doctor discovers a mass or peculiar calcifications on a screening mammogram, or a lump or nodule in the breast at some point during a medical or self-examination. Less commonly, a man or woman might note a red or swollen breast or a mass or nodule below the arm.

The following exams may also be used to diagnose breast cancers or for follow-up checking out after a breast cancer diagnosis.

Imaging Tests.

Imaging assessments show pictures of the inner part of the body. They can show if most cancers have spread. The following imaging tests of the breast can also be achieved to learn extra about a suspicious location found in the breast at some stage in screening. In addition to these, different new kinds of tests are being studied.

Diagnostic Mammography.

Diagnostic mammography is similar to screening mammography without that more pics of the breast are taken. It is regularly used when an individual is experiencing signs, such as a new lump or nipple discharge. Diagnostic mammography may additionally be used if something suspicious is located on a screening mammogram.

Ultrasound.

Ultrasound makes use of sound waves to create a picture of the breast tissue. An ultrasound can distinguish between a strong mass, which might also be cancer, and a fluid-filled cyst, which is typically no longer cancer.

Magnetic Resonance Imaging (MRI). An MRI uses magnetic fields, no longer x-rays, to produce exact pix of the body. A unique dye known as a distinction medium is given earlier than the scan to help create a clear photograph of feasible cancer. This dye is injected into the patient's vein. A breast MRI may be used after a character has been identified with cancer to discover how a good deal the disease has grown throughout the breast or to take a look at the different breasts for cancer.

Breast MRI might also be a screening option, alongside mammography, for any person with a very excessive threat of creating breast cancer and for some girls who have a history of breast cancer. MRI may additionally be used if locally superior breast cancers are diagnosed or if chemotherapy or endocrine remedy is being given first, accompanied by using a repeated MRI for surgical planning (see Types of Treatment). Finally, MRI may also be used as a surveillance approach following breast cancer prognosis and treatment.

Biopsy.

A biopsy is the elimination of a small quantity of tissue for examination beneath a microscope. Other tests can propose that most cancers are present, but only a biopsy can make a particular diagnosis. A pathologist then analyzes the sample(s). A pathologist is a doctor who specializes in interpreting laboratory checks and evaluating cells, tissues, and organs to diagnose disease. There are one-of-a-kind kinds of biopsies, categorized via the approach and/or size of the needle used to acquire the tissue sample.

Fine needle aspiration biopsy. This kind of biopsy uses a skinny needle to eliminate a small sample of cells.

Core Needle Biopsy.

This type of biopsy uses a wider needle to remove a large pattern of tissue. This is typically the desired biopsy technique. If a tumor is identified, most cancer biomarkers, such as hormone receptor reputation (ER, PR) and HER2 status, will be tested to help guide therapy options. These biomarkers are located on the tumor cells.

Additional kinds of biomarkers can be found in the blood or different fluids, even though these are no longer usually used to set up a breast cancer diagnosis. They are made by using the tumor or through the body in response to cancer. This information will assist the doctor to endorse a therapy plan. Local anesthesia, which is medicine to block pain, is used to reduce the patient's soreness during the procedure.

Surgical Biopsy.

This type of biopsy removes the greatest amount of tissue. Because the surgical procedure is first-rate achieved after a cancer prognosis has been made, a surgical biopsy is generally no longer the advocated way to diagnose breast cancer. Most often, non-surgical core needle biopsies are recommended to diagnose breast cancer to restrict the quantity of tissue removed. Since many humans who are encouraged to bear breast biopsy are not recognized with cancer, the use of a needle biopsy for analysis reduces the number of people who have surgery unnecessarily.

Image-guided Biopsy.
During this procedure, a needle is guided to the region of the mass or calcifications with the help of an imaging technique, such as mammography, ultrasound, or MRI. These are usually core needle biopsies, but they can also be exceptional needle aspiration biopsies. A stereotactic biopsy is a type of image-guided biopsy that is performed with the use of mammography to assist guide the needle.

Your medical doctor will let you be aware of what kind of biopsy is first-rate for your situation. A small steel clip is commonly put into the breast at the time of biopsy to mark the place the biopsy pattern was taken, in case the tissue is cancerous and an extra surgical procedure is needed. This clip is normally titanium, so it will not cause trouble with future imaging tests, but check with your medical doctor earlier than you have any imaging assessments done.

Sentinel Lymph Node Biopsy.

When most cancers spread through the lymphatic system, the lymph node or group of lymph nodes that most cancers reach first is known as the "sentinel" lymph node. In breast cancer, these are typically the lymph nodes under the hands known as the axillary lymph nodes. The sentinel lymph node biopsy process is a way to find out if there is cancer in the lymph nodes close to the breast. Learn more about sentinel lymph node biopsy in the Types of Treatment section.

Analyzing The Biopsy Sample

Analyzing the sample(s) eliminated in the course of the biopsy can assist your doctor research specific points of most cancers that help decide your therapy options.

Tumor Features.

Examination of the tumor below the microscope is used to decide if it is invasive or non-invasive (in situ); ductal, lobular, or any other type of breast cancer; and whether most cancers have spread to the lymph nodes. The margins or edges of the tumor are also examined, and the distance from the tumor to the edge of the tissue that was removed is measured, which is known as margin width.

Estrogen Receptors (ER) And Progesterone Receptors (PR).

Testing for ER and PR helps determine both the patient's hazard of recurrence (risk of most cancers coming back) and the kind of therapy that is most in all likelihood to decrease the risk of recurrence. Generally, hormonal therapy, also called endocrine remedy or hormone-blocking therapy, reduces the chance of recurrence of ER-positive and/or PR-positive cancers.

Guidelines endorse that the ER and PR repute should be tested on the breast tumor and/or areas of spread for everybody newly recognized with invasive breast most cancers or when there is a breast most cancers recurrence. For those with ductal carcinoma in situ (DCIS), testing for ER reputation is recommended to discover if hormone therapy may additionally limit the threat of future breast cancer.

Human Epidermal Boom Aspect Receptor 2 (HER2).

The HER2 fame of cancer helps determine whether drugs that target the HER2 receptor, such as trastuzumab (Herceptin) and pertuzumab (Perjeta), would possibly help deal with cancer. This check is solely performed on invasive cancers. Guidelines advise that HER2 testing be carried out when you are first recognized with invasive breast cancer. In addition, if cancer has spread to another part of your physique or comes lower back after treatment, testing has to be carried out again on the new tumor or areas where the most cancers have spread.

HER2 checks are commonly sincerely nice or negative, which means that your cancer has either a high or low degree of HER2. If you take a look at the consequences that are no longer, in reality, tremendous or negative, extra checking may be done, both on a unique tumor pattern or with a distinctive test. Sometimes, even with repeated testing, the outcomes may additionally not be conclusive, so you and your health practitioner will have to talk about the best therapy option.

If the cancer is HER2 positive, HER2-targeted therapy may also be an advocated therapy alternative for you.

Grade.

The tumor grade is also decided from a biopsy. Grade refers to how exclusive the cancer cells look from healthful cells and whether they show up slower developing or quicker growing. If cancer appears similar to healthful tissue and has special phone groupings, it is called "well-differentiated" or a "low-grade tumor." If the cancerous tissue looks very special from healthy tissue, it is called "poorly differentiated" or a "high-grade tumor." There are three grades: grade 1 (well differentiated), grade 2 (moderately differentiated), and grade three (poorly differentiated).

CHAPTER 8

TREATMENT OF BREAST CANCER

The important treatments for breast most cancers are:

- Surgery
- Radiotherapy
- Chemotherapy
- Hormone therapy
- Targeted therapy

You may additionally have one of these treatments or a combination. The kind of aggregate of treatments you have will depend on how the cancer was recognized and the stage it is at.

Breast cancer recognized at routine screening may additionally be at an early stage, however,

breast cancer identified when you have signs
may also be at a later stage and require
exceptional treatment.

Your MTD ought to discuss with you which
treatments are most suitable.

Choosing the right treatment for you
When figuring out what remedy is first-class for
you, your medical doctors will consider:

- The stage and grade of most cancers (how
  large it is and how ways it has spread)
- Your everyday health
- Whether you have experienced the
  menopause
- You should be in a position to talk about
  your treatment with your care crew at any
  time and ask questions.

Treatment Overview.
Surgery is generally the first type of cure for
breast cancer. The type of surgical operation you

have will depend on the kind of breast cancer you have.

Surgery is generally observed via chemotherapy or radiotherapy or, in some cases, hormone or targeted therapies.

Again, the therapy you may have will rely on the type of breast cancer.

Your doctor will discuss the most suitable treatment layout with you. Chemotherapy or hormone therapy will on occasion be the first treatment.

Secondary Breast Cancer.
Most breast cancers are determined at an early stage. But a small share of girls find out they have breast cancer after it's unfolded to other parts of the body (metastasis).

If this is the case, the type of cure you have can also be different. Secondary cancer, also referred to as "advanced" or "metastatic" cancer, is now not curable.

Treatment pursuits to attain remission, where cancer shrinks or disappears, and you sense every day and can experience existence to the full.

Surgery.
There are 2 main types of breast most cancers surgery:

- Breast-conserving surgery, where the cancerous lump (tumor) is removed
- Mastectomy, the place the entire breast is removed
- In many cases, a mastectomy can be accompanied by a reconstructive surgical operation to try to recreate a breast.

Studies have shown that breast-conserving surgical treatment followed by way of radiotherapy is as successful as complete mastectomy at treating early-stage breast cancer.

Breast-conserving Surgery.
Breast-conserving surgical procedure levels
from a lumpectomy or large local excision,
where the tumor and a little surrounding breast
tissue are removed, to a partial mastectomy or
quadrantectomy, where up to a quarter of the
breast is removed.

If you have breast-conserving surgery, the
amount of breast tissue that is removed will
depend on:

- The type of cancer you have
- The size of the tumor and the place it is in
  your breast
- The amount of surrounding tissue that
  needs to be removed
- The measurement of your breasts

Your doctor will continually cast off an area of
healthy breast tissue around the tumor, which
will be tested for traces of cancer.

- If there's no cancer present in the healthy tissue, there is much less risk that cancer will return.
- If cancer cells are discovered in the surrounding tissue, extra tissue might also want to be eliminated from your breast.

After having breast-conserving surgery, you will commonly be supplied radiotherapy to ruin any last cancer cells.

Mastectomy.
A mastectomy is the elimination of all the breast tissue, together with the nipple.

If there are no apparent signs and symptoms that most cancers have to unfold to your lymph nodes, you may also have a mastectomy, where your breast is removed, along with a sentinel lymph node biopsy.

If most cancers have spread to your lymph nodes, you will likely want greater giant elimination (clearance) of lymph nodes from the region underneath your arm (axilla).

Reconstruction.
Breast reconstruction is surgery to make a new breast shape that appears as plentiful as possible like your other breast.

Reconstruction can be finished at the same time as a mastectomy (immediate reconstruction), or it can be achieved later (delayed reconstruction).

It can be performed both via inserting a breast implant or with the aid of the usage of tissue from some other phase of your body to create a new breast.

Lymph Node Surgery.
To locate if cancer has spread, a manner referred to as a sentinel lymph node biopsy may also be done.

The sentinel lymph nodes are the first lymph nodes that most cancer cells reach if they spread.

They're sections of the lymph nodes beneath your fingers (axillary lymph nodes).

The position of the sentinel lymph nodes varies, so they're recognized by the use of a combination of a radioisotope and a blue dye.

The sentinel lymph nodes are examined in the laboratory to see if there are any cancer cells present. This offers a proper indicator of whether most cancers have spread.

If there are most cancer cells in the sentinel nodes, you may additionally need in addition surgical treatment to remove greater lymph nodes from below your arm.

Radiotherapy.
Radiotherapy uses managed doses of radiation to kill most cancer cells. It's generally given after surgical treatment and chemotherapy to kill any remaining cancer cells.

If you want radiotherapy, your cure will start about a month after your surgical treatment or chemotherapy to supply your physique with a chance to recover.

You'll possibly have radiotherapy classes three to 5 days a week, for three to 5 weeks. Each session will remain for a few minutes.

The Types Of Radiotherapy.
The type of radiotherapy you have will rely on the type of breast cancer and the type of surgical treatment you have. Some females may no longer want to have radiotherapy at all.

Types of radiotherapy include:

- Breast radiotherapy – after breast-conserving surgery, radiation is utilized to complete of the closing breast tissue
- Chest-wall radiotherapy – after a mastectomy, radiotherapy is utilized on the chest wall

- Breast raise – some girls may additionally be supplied an improvement of high-dose radiotherapy in the vicinity where most cancers used to be removed; however, this might also affect the appearance of your breast, especially if you have massive breasts, and can once in a while have different facet effects, which includes hardening of breast tissue (fibrosis)
- Radiotherapy to the lymph nodes – where radiotherapy is aimed at the armpit (axilla) and the surrounding vicinity to kill any cancer that may also be in the lymph nodes

The aspect outcomes of radiotherapy
Side effects of radiotherapy include:

- Irritation and darkening of the skin on your breast, which can also lead to sore, red, weepy skin
- Extreme tiredness (fatigue)
- Excess fluid build-up in your arm precipitated by using blockage of the

lymph nodes underneath your arm
(lymphoedema)

Chemotherapy.
Chemotherapy involves using an anti-cancer
(cytotoxic) medicinal drug to kill cancer cells.

It's normally used after surgical treatment to
destroy any cancer cells that have no longer been
removed. This is called adjuvant chemotherapy.

In some cases, you may additionally have
chemotherapy earlier than surgery, which is
frequently used to cut back a massive tumor.
This is called neoadjuvant chemotherapy.

Several unique drug treatments are used in
chemotherapy, and 2 to 3 are often given at once.

The desire for medication and the aggregate will
rely on the kind of breast cancer you have and
how far it has spread.

Chemotherapy is usually given as an outpatient treatment, which means you will no longer have to continue to be in a health facility overnight.

The medicines are usually given through a drip straight into a vein.

In some cases, you may also be given tablets that you can take at home. You may additionally have chemotherapy sessions as soon as each two to four weeks and then have a break. Each remedy session is regarded as a cycle. You may also have up to 8 cycles of chemotherapy.

The important side results of chemotherapy are caused by its impact on normal, healthful cells, such as immune cells.

Side consequences of chemotherapy include:

- Infections
- Loss of appetite
- Feeling sick
- Being sick

- Tiredness
- Hair loss
- Sore mouth

Many facet outcomes can be avoided or controlled with medicines that your health practitioner can prescribe.

Chemotherapy medication can additionally stop the manufacturing of estrogen in your body, which is acknowledged to motivate the boom of some breast cancers.

If you have no longer experienced menopause, your periods may give up whilst you are having chemotherapy treatment.

After you have finished the direction of chemotherapy, your ovaries ought to begin producing estrogen again.

But this does no longer always occur and you may additionally enter early menopause. This is extra likely in girls over 40, as they're closer to menopausal age.

Your doctor will discuss with you the effect that therapy will have on your fertility.

Chemotherapy For Secondary Breast Cancer.
If your breast cancer has to unfold beyond the breast and lymph nodes to different parts of your body, chemotherapy will not remedy cancer, however, it may additionally reduce the tumor, relieve your symptoms and help prolong your life.

Hormone Treatment.
Some breast cancers are inspired to develop by using the hormones estrogen or progesterone, which are found naturally in your body. These are regarded as hormone receptor-positive cancers.

Hormone remedy lowers the degrees of estrogen or progesterone hormones in your body or stops their effects.

The type of hormone remedy you have will depend on the stage and grade of cancer, which hormone it is touchy to, your age, whether you have experienced menopause, and what other kind of treatment you are having.

You'll likely have hormone therapy after surgical operation and chemotherapy, but it's on occasion given before the surgical treatment to reduce a tumor and make it less complicated to remove.

Hormone remedies may additionally be used as the sole therapy for breast cancer if your conventional fitness prevents you from having surgery, chemotherapy, or radiotherapy.

In most cases, you may need to take hormone therapy for 5 years or more after having surgery.

If the type of breast most cancers you have is not sensitive to hormones, hormone remedy will have no effect.

Tamoxifen.
Tamoxifen stops estrogen from binding to estrogen-receptor-positive most cancer cells. It's taken each day as a pill or liquid.

Aromatase Inhibitors.
If you have skilled menopause, you might also be presented with an aromatase inhibitor.

- This type of remedy blocks aromatase, a substance that helps the body to produce estrogen after menopause. Before menopause, estrogen is made through the ovaries.

- 3 aromatase inhibitors may be offered. These are anastrozole, exemestane and letrozole. These are taken as a tablet once a day.

- Ovarian ablation or suppression
- In women who have not skilled menopause, estrogen is produced via the ovaries.

- Ovarian ablation or suppression stops the ovaries from working and producing estrogen.

- Ablation can be achieved using surgical treatment or radiotherapy. It permanently stops the ovaries from working and the ability to ride menopause early.

- Ovarian suppression involves using a medicine called goserelin, which is a luteinizing hormone-releasing hormone agonist (LHRHa).

- Your durations will give up while you are taking it, although they have to begin again once your remedy is complete.

- If you're drawing near menopause (around the age of 50), your durations may no longer start again after you cease taking goserelin.

- Goserelin comes as an injection you have as soon as a month.

Targeted Therapies.
Targeted healing procedures are drugs that change the way cells work and assist to stop cancer from developing and spreading. Not all kinds of breast cancers can be treated with centered therapies

The focused therapy most often used to treat breast cancer is trastuzumab (also recognized via the manufacturer's identified Herceptin).

Another focused therapy known as abemaciclib (also regarded by way of the manufacturer Verzenios) can be used to deal with certain types of breast cancer. You might also be supplied it if most cancers have spread to other components of your body or it's probably to come back. It's given alongside hormone therapy.

Some centered treatment plans are given through a drip into a vein. Others come as tablets.

Side effects of targeted cures include:

- Shivering and feeling unwell
- Diarrhea
- Beeling and being sick
- Headache
- Cough
- Skin rash

Bisphosphonates.
If you have been via menopause, you may be provided bisphosphonates (zoledronic acid or sodium clodronate).

Recent research has shown they may assist to minimize the danger of breast cancers spreading to your bones and somewhere else in your body.

Bisphosphonates will in all likelihood be given to you at an equal time as chemotherapy, either immediately into a vein or as tablets.

Rarely, they can motivate kidney issues and osteonecrosis of the jaw (when a bone in the jaw dies).

Your doctor will explain the benefits and possible aspect outcomes before beginning this treatment.

CHAPTER 9

COMPLICATIONS OF BREAST CANCER TREATMENTS

Treatment for breast cancer can result in damaging facets or problems for all people who are going through it. For example, the use of chemotherapy tablets comes with a range of side effects. How your physique reacts to a remedy plan, however, can be extraordinary from anybody else. It all relies upon the kind of breast cancer treatment being administered to you. Talk to your physician if you have any side outcomes or problems while being treated for breast cancer.

Chemotherapy.
Chemotherapy attacks swiftly dividing cells. Cancer cells, alongside skin cells, and digestive tract cells are the most susceptible to

chemotherapy medication. This can lead to hair loss, nausea, and vomiting. Doctors regularly will prescribe you additional medicines at some point during chemotherapy to reduce or relieve nausea and vomiting. Other side effects include:

- Infection
- Fatigue
- Bruising
- Bleeding
- Sleep disturbances

Many of these aspects' consequences can be attributed to low blood counts. This is a common prevalence at some stage in chemotherapy because the dividing blood cells in the bone marrow are additionally inclined to harm from medicines used in this type of treatment. In uncommon cases, some chemotherapy tablets can cause coronary heart damage or set off most cancers such as leukemia.

Chemotherapy in premenopausal ladies may also harm ovaries to the factor that they end up producing hormones. This can cause early menopausal signs and symptoms such as vaginal dryness and warm flashes. Menstrual periods may also give up or emerge as irregular. Getting pregnant may additionally also end up difficult. Women who's journey chemotherapy-caused menopause may additionally also face a higher hazard of osteoporosis.

Most people find that side consequences go away after the remedy is finished. However, the emotional distress of the ride might also motivate the bodily side results to sense greater intensity. Some may have troubles with awareness and reminiscence loss, recognized as "chemo-brain," "chemo-fog," or "chemo-memory." This is typically short-lived.

Psychological side consequences of chemotherapy and breast most cancers also include:

- Depression
- Fear

- Sadness
- Feelings of isolation
- Sleep disturbances

Some people have a difficult time readjusting to the way of life they had before treatment. Thoughts of a relapse can be daunting. Talking with a therapist, support groups, or ordinary contact with a loved one for the duration of this period is recommended.

Radiation Therapy.
Radiation therapy can result in more serious side effects. These can boost slowly. But over time, the facet effects, which at first, seemed manageable can come to be debilitating. Serious complications include:

- Inflamed lung tissue
- Heart damage
- Secondary cancers

These side outcomes are very rare. More common however much less serious ones encompass skin burns, inflammation or discoloration, fatigue, and lymphedema.

Hormone Therapy.

Some kinds of hormone therapy decrease estrogen levels in women and increase the chance of osteoporosis. Your medical doctor may additionally display your bone mineral density whilst you're taking this medication. Lower estrogen degrees additionally may lead to vaginal dryness and irritation. Other types of hormonal therapy amplify your hazard of blood clots and endometrial cancer.

Mastectomy.

A mastectomy is the surgical removal of all or part of the breast. According to Johns Hopkins Medicine, issues include:

- Temporary swelling of the breast
- Breast tenderness
- Hardness due to scar tissue that can shape the web site of the incision
- Wound contamination or bleeding

- Swelling of the arm due to lymph node removal, referred to as lymphedema
- Phantom breast pain, including signs such as disagreeable itching, a sensation of "pins and needles," pressure, and throbbing

A mastectomy also has psychological implications. Some ladies may locate it distressing to lose one or each breast. You might also experience melancholy or anxiousness following the surgery. It's vital to tackle these feelings thru therapy, an assistant group, or different means.

You may pick to have reconstructive breast surgery following a mastectomy to maintain the same physical appearance before the procedure. Others may additionally pick to use breast prostheses to acquire the same results.

But most of these treatments do not simply affect cancer cells. They additionally can affect wholesome cells and can exchange how you feel. This ought to motivate a wide variety of aspect consequences including:

Loss Of Appetite.

Radiation, chemo, immunotherapy, some hormonal therapies, and even some ache meds can make you much less hungry and lead to loss of appetite or taste, all of which can make it difficult to get the nutrition you need.

Try these hints to make certain you're eating a wholesome diet:

- Eat a few small foods for the day as an alternative to three massive ones.
- Try an "instant breakfast" combination or other nutritional shakes between meals.
- Eat your greatest meal of the day when you are most hungry.
- Drink water or other liquids either a 1/2 hour earlier than or after meals so they don't make you too full.
- Prepare foods that are colorful and appealing to the eyes.

- Try reasonable exercising to make your appetite bigger, as long as your medical doctor says it's OK.

The non-surgical breast cancer remedy's goal is to destroy cancer cells. These treatments include:

- Chemotherapy
- Radiation
- Hormone therapies
- Immunotherapies (sometimes known as organic therapies)
- Targeted therapies

But most of these remedies don't affect simply most cancer cells. They also can affect healthful cells and can change how you feel. This should purpose many facet effects including:

- Loss of appetite
- Nausea and vomiting
- Weakness and fatigue
- Mouth sores or dry mouth

- Taste adjustments from most cancers or chemo treatments
- Hair loss
- Weight gain
- Early menopause
- A greater hazard of infections
- Bleeding
- Diarrhea

Medications and other cures that address these consequences can assist ease many of these aspects' effects.

Nausea and Vomiting.

Chemo, radiation, centered therapy, and immunotherapy can cause nausea now and then vomiting. But localized radiation for breast cancer is less likely to cause vomiting. It can occur right after the remedy or a few days later. Ask your health practitioner about medicines that can make you sense better. Also, hold track of when you're nauseated. You may be able to spot patterns that can help you get beforehand of the problem. Also:

- Eat small ingredients extra often and keep away from greasy ingredients and citrus.
- Try meals at room temperature as an alternative to very warm or cold.
- When you're nauseated, try bland ingredients like crackers, gelatin, ice chips, rice, plain mashed potatoes, or applesauce.
- Avoid smells that bother you while you are eating.

Call your health practitioner if you have severe nausea or you're vomiting a lot. If you throw up, wait an hour earlier than you eat or drink anything. Then, start with ice chips and gradually add food. Chamomile, ginger root tea, or ginger ale can sometimes assist settle your stomach.

Weakness And Fatigue.

Weakness is when you're no longer as sturdy as you have been before, or now not as sturdy as you need to be for primary everyday tasks.

Chemo, hormone therapies, some targeted therapies, and some pain meds should target weakness.

Cancer-related fatigue is a distressing and relentless state that has a vast effect on your capability to function. You don't have the strength to do what you need to do or you feel worn out all the time, even when there's no apparent motive for it. The fatigue is out of proportion to your exercise level. Cancer itself or chemo, radiation, hormonal, immunotherapy, and targeted treatment options can cause fatigue.

Work with your physician to regulate your way of life to locate approaches that can hold weak spots and fatigue to a minimum. Some suitable policies of thumb include:

- Make sure you get ample rest. Sleep at least 7 hours a night, and strive to lie down during the day to rest if you're nevertheless tired. Avoid caffeine late in the day.

- Exercise. Short walks can provide you with greater energy. If you're more active, you'll rest better.
- Save your energy for the things that are genuinely necessary to you. Get help from households and buddies with errands and different chores.
- If you sense pain, let your health practitioner know. There is nearly always redress that can help.
- Eat plenty of iron-rich foods like lean meat, beans, dark, leafy vegetables, and iron-fortified cereals or pasta.

If your body has too few crimson blood cells, a situation called anemia, your physician can also advocate erythropoietin or darbepoetin, treatments that stimulate the bone marrow to make purple blood cells. You can get them by injection, which you can once in a while do on your own at home. If you get this treatment, your health practitioner will watch you to see if you have rashes, allergic reactions, and problems with blood pressure.

Mouth Soreness.

Chemo, radiation, and some centered treatment plans can make your mouth and throat sore. You may even be aware of sores, or "ulcers," that can be red and swollen. This is referred to as mucositis. Check with your doctor or dentist to see what can stop your pain. Some options include:

- Ask your physician about drugs to ease mouth soreness.
- Choose soft foods that won't irritate your mouth, such as scrambled eggs, macaroni and cheese, pureed cooked vegetables, and bananas.
- Cut food into small pieces.
- Avoid citrus fruits, spicy or salty items, and hard foods.
- Avoid very bloodless or warm beverages
- Hair Loss

Breast cancer redress that may want to cause hair loss consists of chemo, radiation, hormonal therapy, and centered therapy.

Not anybody will lose their hair at some stage in cancer treatment. It depends on the kind of remedy and the dose. Your medical doctor can inform you if you can assume hair loss. Talk to them. It helps to know what to expect.

While some women will observe their hair becoming thinner, others will lose it completely, inclusive of eyelashes and eyebrows, pubic hair, and arm and leg hair. Sometimes it happens suddenly, or you may additionally have a greater gradual loss a few weeks after you begin treatment. Some people use cooling caps to assist limit hair loss due to chemotherapy. Cooling the scalp before, during, and after can also limit the quantity of chemo that gets into hair follicles. Since there are some long-term protection issues with the use of cooling caps, it is nice to speak with your physician before deciding to use one.

Some women prepare by getting a brief hair fashion before chemotherapy begins. You can additionally strive for hair wraps and wigs.

When hair grows back, the texture may additionally be different, but many girls won't observe any changes. The appropriate news about hair loss from chemotherapy is that it stops as soon as therapy is over. After a few months, hair can regrow completely.

Hormone Therapy.
You may word a bit of hair thinning or hair loss, usually in the front or center phase of the head. Hormone therapies work by lowering estrogen levels, but scientists don't know exactly why they lead to hair loss. It typically takes from 6 months to two years to note hair loss from hormone therapy. It might go away after 12 months or so, but thinning regularly lasts for as long as you take the medication. The outcomes cease a few months after you end up taking the medication.

Targeted Breast Cancer Therapy.

These medications, including palbociclib (Ibrance), pertuzumab (Perjeta), and ribociclib (Kisqali) may additionally cause hair loss in some people. You'll note it properly away and your hair won't start to grow again till countless months after you cease taking these medications.

Immunotherapy.

In very uncommon cases, immunotherapy can also cause hair loss in some people. Some examples are pembrolizumab (Keytruda) and dostarlimab-gxly (Jemperli).

Radiation.

Radiation solely reasons hair loss in the specific part of the body it targets. This may also be the nipple or armpit if you have hair there. But it can also additionally be the head of your breast most cancers have spread to components of your head like the brain.

May motivate pain, burning, swelling, and skin discoloration (typically red) at the website of radiation (often the breast). There may additionally even be blistering or peeling of the skin. In uncommon cases, the radiation can also burn a bit of the lung and cause it to swell (pneumonitis). The risk adjustments depend on the size of the location that receives radiation. And the swelling in the lung tissue tends to go away with time.

Weight Gain.

Breast most cancers remedies like the chemo drug ixabepilone (Ixempra) and the targeted remedy drug bevacizumab (Avastin) alongside a wide variety of hormone therapy treatments or steroids given with chemo can lead you to put on some kilos in the course of breast cancer treatment.

If you note you are gaining weight, let your doctor be aware of it and see what they assume would possibly assist you. Don't go on a weight loss program on your personal -- your body wishes for a lot of vitamins at some stage in breast cancer treatment.

Higher Risk Of Infections.
Many breast cancer cures can weaken your immune device and elevate your danger of infection. Common areas for infection include:

- Lungs
- Mouth
- Throat
- Sinuses
- Skin

Chemotherapy and radiation remedy for breast cancer can minimize the number of white blood cells your physique makes. Those cells battle infections. Try to continue to be out of large crowds and away from unwell adults and adolescents for 7 to 10 days after you have chemotherapy. That's when you commonly have the fewest white blood cells.

Contact your health practitioner properly if you get sick. You would possibly notice:

- Colored mucus in saliva or nasal drainage
- Fever of 100.5 degrees F or higher
- Sore or burning throat
- Swelling, redness, warmth, or pus at the damaged site
- Cough or shortness of breath
- Your health practitioner may suggest antibiotics as a precaution. Or they may propose you get a flu shot before you start chemotherapy.

If your white blood telephone counts are too low, your doctor may additionally provide you a cure called G-CSF (granulocyte colony-stimulating aspect -- Neulasta or Neupogen) or GM-CSF (granulocyte-macrophage colony-stimulating thing -- Leukine).

Infertility.
Some breast cancer treatments can make you infertile for a while. In some cases, remedies

should make you infertile forever. The impact relies upon in phase on how lengthy you're on treatment, the dosage, your age, and other factors.

Here are some approaches that most cancers remedies can affect your fertility:

- Chemotherapy may also decrease the number of eggs your physique releases to be fertilized.
- Radiation can also damage your ovaries and uterus.
- Hormone therapy might also interrupt your menstrual cycles and make it tougher to conceive.
- If you think you might desire to get pregnant after most cancers are done, speak with your medical doctor about fertility protection methods, such as accumulating eggs to freeze for later use.

Brain Fog.

Some humans call this "chemo brain." But you can have this frequent type of mental fog even without chemotherapy, or from different cancers such as radiation, immunotherapy, and hormone therapy. You can also word problems for the duration of and after your treatments. There is no proof that these cognitive troubles lead to dementia. Symptoms may also include:

- Forgetfulness
- Trouble concentrating
- Mild memory loss, such as names and dates
- Difficulty multitasking
- These problems commonly go away within 6-12 months after your remedy ends. But some human beings may additionally have cognitive issues for years.

Emotional Impact.

Cancer remedies can affect you mentally as well as physically. For example, some remedies can set off inflammatory immune reactions that may additionally lead to depression, anxiety, and other temper changes. You might also feel:

- Irritable
- Worried
- Unmotivated
- Uninterested in intercourse or different activities
- Hopeless
- Anxious

Cancer can be a life-changing diagnosis. Many people have instances when they feel overwhelmed emotionally or mentally by it. Talk to your doctor so you can determine if the signs stem from your treatments. Different types of psychotherapy and mental health counseling may also assist you to get through this time.

Other Side Effects of Breast Cancer Treatment.

Different humans can have distinctive responses to identical breast cancer treatments. That's why it's important to tell your healthcare team about all of your reactions. Some facet results you would possibly prefer to appear out for that are no longer listed above include:

Chemotherapy.
May purpose digestive problems (diarrhea, constipation), tingling, numbness, pain, skipped periods, or early menopause. Your health practitioner may be capable to remedy many of these aspects' consequences with supportive medications.

Hormone Therapy.
The drug tamoxifen, which blocks estrogen from attaching to cancer cells, can lead to hot flashes and vaginal dryness, discharge, or bleeding. It may also additionally be linked in very uncommon instances to cataracts, blood clots, and uterine cancer.

A comparable crew of tablets known as aromatase inhibitors, or AIs, may additionally cause warm flashes, vaginal dryness, and muscle and joint pain. They additionally could elevate your hazard of osteoporosis and broken bones. In uncommon cases, scientists have linked them to thinning hair and greater cholesterol. Some AI meds seem to have fewer facet effects for one-of-a-kind women, though it's no longer clear why. So ask your medical doctor if switching might assist with your facet effects.

Immunotherapy.
Immunotherapy capsules may additionally cause flu-like symptoms -- fever, chills, body aches, sore throat, runny nose -- and GI issues like diarrhea.

When Are Side Effects an Emergency?
Call your nurse or health practitioner if you have:

- A temperature over 100.4 F. If you have any fever or chills, inform your physician properly. If you can't get in touch with your doctor, go to the emergency room.
- New mouth sores, patches, a swollen tongue, or bleeding gums

- A dry, burning, scratchy, or "swollen" throat
- A cough that is new or doesn't go away
- Changes in how your bladder works, which includes a need to go urgently or greater often, burning when you pee, or blood in your urine
- Digestive modifications, inclusive of heartburn; nausea, vomiting, constipation, or diarrhea that is severe or lasts longer than 2 or 3 days; or blood in your stools.

CHAPTER 10

FOODS THAT PREVENT BREAST CANCER

A woman can also restrict her hazard for breast cancer by eating greater portions of ingredients with vitamins and antioxidants confirmed to war cancer.

Certain nutritional vitamins and vitamins can limit your threat of breast cancer. If you meet breast cancer threat factors, devour the following 11 healthful substances to lower your risk.

1. Dark Leafy Greens

Kale, spinach, and collard veggies are some of the many dark, leafy veggies that can fight breast cancer. Leafy greens get loaded with antioxidants that can smash free radicals that cause cancer.

Dark leafy vegetables go tremendously with almost every meal. Sautee them in garlic and olive oil, or add them to salads and sandwiches. They also style extremely well in soups and chilis.

Dark leafy veggies include:

- Arugula
- Bok choy
- Collard greens
- Dandelion greens
- Kale
- Mustard greens
- Spinach
- Swiss chard
- Turnip greens

2. Berries

Berries include antioxidants and dietary nutritional vitamins that can guard cells, restore broken cells, and slow the unfolding of most cancer cells. Darker berries have 50% extra antioxidants than lighter berries.

Berries go fantastic with cereal, Greek yogurt, and oatmeal. They can also get fruit salads. Choose glowing berries over dehydrated berries, as the latter usually include delivered sugars and fewer nutrients.

Berries include:

- Blackberries
- Blueberries
- Boysenberries
- Cranberries
- Elderberries
- Lingonberries
- Raspberries
- Strawberries

3. Citrus Fruits

Citrus fruits incorporate eating regimen C, folate, calcium, and many distinct nutritional vitamins that may additionally forestall and combat breast cancer.

Citrus fruits can be eaten undeniably as a snack between meals. They can additionally embellish the taste of tea and water. Try the use of citrus fruits as an ingredient in salsas, marinades, salads, and healthful desserts.

Citrus fruits include:

- Clementines
- Grapefruits
- Kumquats
- Lemons
- Limes
- Oranges
- Pomelos
- Tangerines
- Tangelos

4. Fermented Foods

Fermented foods are immoderate in probiotics, which remain "healthy" microorganisms and yeasts. Probiotics are right for your digestion. They can additionally forestall your physique from absorbing dangerous toxins that cause breast cancer.

- Apple cider vinegar
- Kefir
- Kimchi
- Kombucha
- Kvass
- Miso
- Natto
- Pickles
- Raw cheese
- Tempeh
- Sauerkraut
- Sourdough bread
- Yogurt

Kefir tastes like a drinkable yogurt. Kombucha is a carbonated drink that contains black tea and natural sugars. Kimchi is a flavorful Korean vegetable dish that accommodates cabbage. Natto is a dish made with fermented soybeans.

Many fermented meals also have antioxidants and nutritional vitamins that can reduce your breast cancer risk. Experiment with many fermented ingredients to locate the ones you like best then begin consuming them regularly.

5. Fatty Fish

Certain varieties of fish include healthful fats and antioxidants that can restrict infection related to breast cancer.

Fatty fish is quality when baked or smoked, and additionally tastes fantastic when used in fish tacos and sandwiches.

Types of healthy fatty fish include:

- Anchovies
- Herring
- Kippers
- Mackerel
- Pilchards
- Salmon

- Sardines
- Trout
- Tuna

6. Allium Veggies

"Allium" is the Latin phrase for garlic. However, there are many extra veggies in the allium household proven to restrict the risk of breast cancer. Allium veggies include excessive amounts of vitamin C and antioxidants. They additionally have sulfurous compounds that can cease blood clots and improve the immune system.

Allium veggies include:

- Chives
- Garlic
- Leeks
- Onions
- Scallions
- Shallots

Allium veggies can get delivered to nearly every meal, especially onions, and garlic. Add these vegetables to stir-fry meals, soups, stews, chilis, and salads.

7. Beans

Beans are a superfood loaded with fiber, vitamins, and many unique nutritional vitamins that ward off breast cancer. The antioxidants in beans can end inflammation and repair broken cells. The nutritional vitamins and minerals in beans can additionally toughen the immune laptop to make you plenty much less prone to illnesses and illnesses like cancer.

Several medical lookups exhibit that women who devour immoderate portions of beans have a minimized risk of breast cancer.

When shopping for beans, keep away from canned beans every time possible. Canned beans usually contain immoderate quantities of sodium and additives. Buy dry beans instead, which can be cooked shortly and with no hassle in a stress cooker. Dry beans are typically low in fee and convenient to shop and hold on hand.

Beans that can decrease your breast most cancers hazard include:

- Black beans
- Chickpeas
- Kidney beans
- Lentils
- Navy beans
- Peas
- Pinto beans
- Soybeans

8. Spices And Herbs

Spices and herbs frequently get used in small quantities to taste meals. However, these components contain excessive quantities of antioxidants, vitamins, and fatty acids that may additionally prevent breast cancer. Plus, they can get introduced to nearly every meal to enlarge its taste and make its dietary value larger.

Turmeric is one of the most daily anti-cancer spices. This spice reduces infection and cell phone damage. The integral anti-cancer agent in turmeric is curcumin. Turmeric is an earthy, peppery spice used in many Indian dishes and curries. This spice can moreover get brought to rice, soups, and tea.

Spices and herbs determined to minimize the threat of breast most cancers include:

- Black pepper
- Cayenne pepper
- Cinnamon
- Ginger
- Oregano
- Rosemary
- Parsley
- Thyme
- Turmeric

9. Cruciferous Veggies

Cruciferous greens are recognized to be a gorgeous cancer-fighting food. After they are chewed and digested, cruciferous veggies shape exceptional compounds that can war and prevent cancer.

These meals can quit cell phone damage, reduce inflammation, and smash the hazardous most cancers cells. They can also deactivate most cancer retailers (cancer-causing substances) and prevent blood vessels from forming internal tumors.

Cruciferous veggies include:

- Arugula
- Bok choy
- Broccoli
- Brussels sprouts
- Cabbage
- Cauliflower
- Collard greens
- Kale
- Radishes
- Rutabaga
- Turnips

- Watercress

Nearly all these veggie styles are notable when introduced to salads and sandwiches, or when served with fish, poultry, and lean meats. They can moreover get delivered to rice bowls, soups, stews, and chilis.

10. Pomegranate

Many lookups show that those pomegranates would possibly additionally cease hostilities with estrogen-dependent cancers, such as breast cancer. Pomegranates contain compounds known as ellagitannins that can end the extent and spread of breast cancer cells.

Drinking pomegranate juice is one of the exceptional and most handy methods to add this fruit to your diet. If you buy complete pomegranates, devour the seeds easily by themselves or add them to salads, oatmeal, yogurt, and smoothies.

11. Green Tea

Green tea carries compounds and various antioxidants that limit a woman's breast cancer risk.

Women who drink at least 10 cups of inexperienced tea may additionally be capable of preventing breast cancer. Green tea can reduce irritation and smash free radicals that cause more than a few types of cancer.

When buying inexperienced tea, choose loose tea leaves or purchase tea bags besides food coloring or specific dangerous additives. Do now no longer buy industrial manufacturers of inexperienced tea with excessive quantities of sugar and artificial flavors that can cancel out the fitness benefits of the tea.

Foods And Liquids To Avoid.
While certain ingredients can additionally protect in opposition to breast cancer, others may additionally enlarge your risk.

As such, it's remarkable to minimize your consumption of the following meals and liquids — or keep away from them altogether:

Alcohol.
Alcohol use, in specific heavy drinking, might also notably enlarge your hazard of breast cancer.

Fast food.
Eating fast meals regularly has many downsides, such as an extended chance of heart disease, diabetes, obesity, and breast cancer.

Fried Foods.
Research indicates that a weight loss design immoderate in fried ingredients might also moreover notably amplify your chance of breast cancer. Indeed, in a study involving 620 Iranian women under 50 years old, fried food consumption used to be the greatest hazard for breast cancer development.

Processed Meats.

Processed meats like bacon and sausage may additionally also expand your risk of breast cancer. A literature evaluation of 18 studies linked particularly processed meat consumption to a 9% elevated breast cancer risk.

Added Sugar.

An eating regimen excessive in introducing sugar might also incredibly expand your risk of breast cancer through the usage of growing contamination and the expression of enzymes associated with most cancers' growth and spread.

Refined Carbs.

Diets high in refined carbs, inclusive of the common Western diet, may additionally increase breast cancer risk. Try changing sophisticated carbs like white bread and sugary baked gadgets with complete grain merchandise and nutrient-dense veggies.

Soy And Breast Cancer.

Many humans are moreover surprised whether soy merchandise — such as tofu, soy milk, and edamame — can have an impact on their risk of breast cancer. Research is mixed.

According to a phase of test-tube and animal studies, eating excessive portions of isoflavones, a compound found in soy, enlarges the chance of breast cancer development. Isoflavones mimic the results of estrogen.

However, research in humans has truly determined that multiplied soy intake is linked to a minimized hazard of growing breast cancer.

What's more, soy intake can also simply improve results and assist defense in opposition to recurrence in human beings diagnosed with breast cancer.

CHAPTER 11

COPING AND SUPPORT

Coping with an analysis of breast cancer can be overwhelming. Find out what you can do, who can help, and how to cope.

Your Feelings.
You would possibly have a range of extraordinary emotions when you're knowledgeable you have cancer. You may additionally feel shocked and upset. You would possibly additionally feel:

- Numb
- Frightened and uncertain
- Confused
- Angry and resentful
- Guilty

You can also additionally have some or all of these feelings. Or you might experience something completely different. Everyone reacts in their way. Sometimes it is difficult to take in the fact that you have most cancers.

Experiencing exclusive emotions is a natural part of coming to phrases with cancer. All varieties of feelings are likely to come and go.

Helping Yourself.
You may additionally be more in a role to cope and make alternatives if you have data about the variety of most cancers and their treatment. The information helps you to be conscious of what to expect.

Taking statistics can be difficult, specifically when you have honestly been diagnosed. Make a list of questions earlier than you see your doctor. Take everyone with you to remind you what you desire to ask. They can additionally aid you to take into account the records that used to be given. Getting a lot of new documents can be an overwhelming trip.

Ask your medical practitioner and nurse experts to explain matters again if you need them to.

Remember that you don't have to sort the entirety out at once. It might also take some time to deal with every issue. Ask for aid if you favor it.

You can also do smart things such as:

- Making lists to help you
- Having a calendar with all appointments
- Having goals
- Planning fun matters spherical weeks that would perchance be trickier than others

Talking To Exclusive People.
Talking to your buddies and spouse and children about your most cancers can aid and assist you. But some human beings are scared of the thoughts they may additionally prefer to deliver

up and won't choose to talk. They may be concerned that you may additionally no longer be in a position to cope with your scenario or be afraid they will say the mistaken thing.

It can stress relationships if your family or pals do not prefer to talk. But speaking to me can help increase trust and guidance between you and them.

Help your family and buddies by way of letting them understand if you would like to discuss what's going on and how you feel.

You would perchance discover it less difficult to talk to anyone outside your non-public pals and family.

Physical Problems.
Breast cancer and its redress are probable to motivate bodily problems. These would perhaps have an impact on the way you experience yourself.

Changes to the structure of one or both breasts and scarring after a surgical operation can have an impact on your self-esteem and how you relate to different people. Some ladies would possibly additionally have some ongoing discomfort and anguish in their breasts after surgery.

Some hormone redress can moreover cause joint and bone pain. Talk to your medical doctor or nurse about this as they can prescribe a medicinal drug to help.

Tiredness and lethargy can be a hassle all through treatment. Resting but also doing some gentle physical challenges can help.

Some redress can cause early menopause and you would perchance have symptoms such as hot flushes and sweats. Your nurse will talk to you about how to cope with the symptoms.

Early menopause additionally functionality that you are no longer in a role to turn out to be pregnant. This can be very challenging to cope with if you had been hoping to have adolescents in the future. Your scientific health practitioner will talk to you about this earlier than your treatment. It's from time to time viable to maintain your eggs or embryos earlier than the remedy starts.

Relationships And Sex.
The physical and emotional adjustments you have would possibly affect your relationships and intercourse life. There are things that you can do to manage this.

Coping Practically.
You and your family may also favor coping with smart matters including:

- Money matters
- Financial support, such as benefits, bad health pay, and grants
- Work issues
- Childcare

Talk to your fitness practitioner or expert nurse to locate who can help. Getting help early with these things can advise that they don't emerge as a large situation later.

Talking To Family, Buddies, And Children.
If you're discovering it tough to cope emotionally, you may additionally prefer to speak to friends or household participants about how you're feeling.

Dealing With Isolation.
Feeling lonely or isolated is very common.

You may additionally feel lonely even when you're surrounded through family and friends. If they haven't experienced most cancers themselves, you may journey like they don't apprehend what you're going through.

Connecting With Human Beings Who Understand.
For some people, connecting with others who are in a comparable state of affairs can help

minimize thoughts of isolation, as well as anxiety or fear.

Survivors may journey through a mixture of feelings, which consists of joy, concern, relief, guilt, and fear. Some people say they admire life more after most cancers are evaluated and have acquired a larger acceptance of themselves. Some humans may additionally decide to put the experience in the back of them and feel that their lives have no longer been modified in an indispensable way.

Others grow to be very anxious about their fitness and are unsure about coping with day-to-day life. Feelings of concern and anxiousness may also nevertheless take place as time passes, then again these ideas no longer be a steady segment of your daily life. If they persist, be positive to speak with a member of your healthcare team.

Survivors may also additionally trip some stress when their typical visits to the fitness care crew give up after finishing treatment. Often, relationships built with the most cancer care groups supply a sense of safety all through treatment, and humans bypass this supply of support. This may also additionally be particularly appropriate when new problems and challenges surface over time, such as any late outcomes of treatment, emotional challenges such as fear of recurrence, sexual health and fertility concerns, and monetary and administrative center issues.

Every survivor has character worries and challenges. With any challenge, an appropriate first step is being capable to apprehend your fears and speak about them. Effective coping requires:

- Understanding the mission you are facing
- Thinking through solutions
- Asking for and allowing the useful resource of others
- Feeling blissful with the course of action you choose

Many survivors discover it useful to be a part of an in-person aid crew or an online regional of survivors. This lets you talk with human beings who have had comparable first-hand experiences. Other picks for finding aid include speaking with a chum or member of your fitness care team, man or girl counseling, or asking for assistance at the mastering beneficial aid center of the place you acquired the treatment.

CONCLUSION

Being diagnosed with breast cancer can affect each day's existence in many ways, depending on what stage it's at and the treatment you will have.

How human beings cope with the prognosis and treatment varies from personality to personality. There are several forms of help available, if you want it.

Forms of information can also include:

- Family and friends, who can be a wonderful useful resource system
- Communicating with other human beings in the same situation
- Finding out as a good deal as viable about your condition

- Not making and striving to do too an entire lot or overexerting yourself
- Making time for yourself.

Doctors and scientists are always searching for higher methods to care for people with breast cancer. To make scientific advances, doctors design lookup research involving volunteers, referred to as clinical trials. Every drug that is now permitted by way of the U.S. Food and Drug Administration (FDA) used to be tested in scientific trials.

Clinical trials are used for all kinds and tiers of breast cancer. Often, scientific trials are a great choice to treat breast cancer. Many focus on new redress to analyze if a new cure is safe, effective, and per danger higher than the current treatments. These kinds of research evaluate new drugs, one-of-a-kind mixtures of treatments, new processes for radiation treatment or surgery, and new techniques of treatment.

People who take part in medical trials can be some of the first to get a remedy before it is handy to the public. However, there are some risks with a scientific trial, inclusive of doable aspect results and the danger that the new remedy may no longer work. People are prompted to talk with their fitness care team about the pros and cons of becoming a member of a special study.

Some clinical trials find out about new approaches to relieve signs and symptoms and aspect outcomes at some point of treatment. Others locate approaches to manipulate the late results that can also appear for a prolonged time after treatment. Talk with your scientific health practitioner about scientific trials for signs and symptoms and side effects.